The Complete Alkaline

Amazing Recipes to Start Your ⌐┐u Boost Your Lifesty

Sam Horton

Table of Contents

RASPBERRIES PANCAKES

Serves: 4

Prep Time: 10 Minutes

Cook Time: 20 Minutes

Total Time: 30 Minutes

INGREDIENTS

- 1 cup whole wheat flour

- ¼ tsp baking soda

- ¼ tsp baking powder

- 1 cup raspberries

- 2 eggs

- 1 cup milk

DIRECTIONS

1. In a bowl combine all ingredients together and mix well

2. In a skillet heat olive oil

3. Pour ¼ of the batter and cook each pancake for 1-2 minutes per side

4. When ready remove from heat and serve

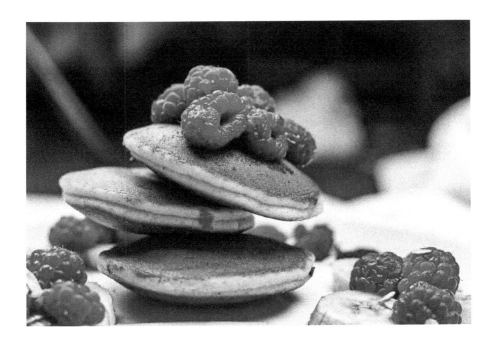

QUINCE PANCAKES

Serves: *4*

Prep Time: *10*   Minutes

Cook Time: *30*   Minutes

Total Time: *40*   Minutes

INGREDIENTS

-         1 cup whole wheat flour

-         ¼ tsp baking soda

-         ¼ tsp baking powder

-         1 cup quince

-         2 eggs

-         1 cup milk

DIRECTIONS

1. In a bowl combine all ingredients together and mix well

2. In a skillet heat olive oil

3. Pour ¼ of the batter and cook each pancake for 1-2 minutes per side

4. When ready remove from heat and serve

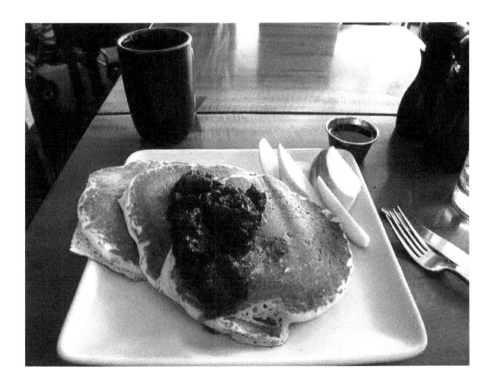

PRUNES PANCAKES

Serves: 4

Prep Time: 10 Minutes

Cook Time: 20 Minutes

Total Time: 30 Minutes

INGREDIENTS

- 1 cup whole wheat flour

- ¼ tsp baking soda

- ¼ tsp baking powder

- 1 cup prunes

- 2 eggs

- 1 cup milk

DIRECTIONS

1. In a bowl combine all ingredients together and mix well

2. In a skillet heat olive oil

3. Pour ¼ of the batter and cook each pancake for 1-2 minutes per side

4. When ready remove from heat and serve

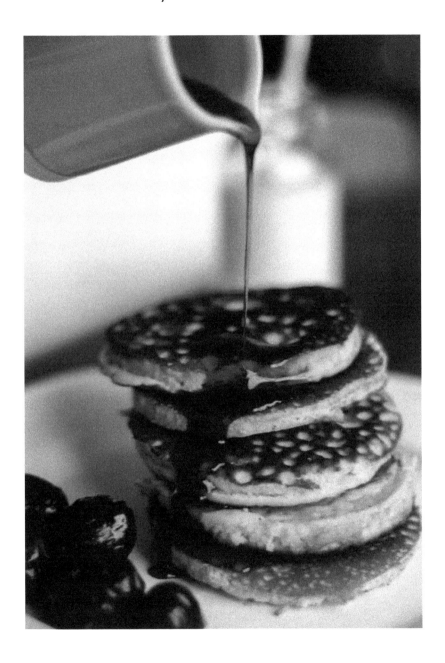

POMEGRANATE PANCAKES

Serves: *4*

Prep Time: *10* Minutes

Cook Time: *20* Minutes

Total Time: *30* Minutes

INGREDIENTS

- 1 cup whole wheat flour

- ¼ tsp baking soda

- ¼ tsp baking powder

- 1 cup pomegranate

- 2 eggs

- 1 cup milk

DIRECTIONS

1. In a bowl combine all ingredients together and mix well

2. In a skillet heat olive oil

3. Pour ¼ of the batter and cook each pancake for 1-2 minutes per side

4. When ready remove from heat and serve

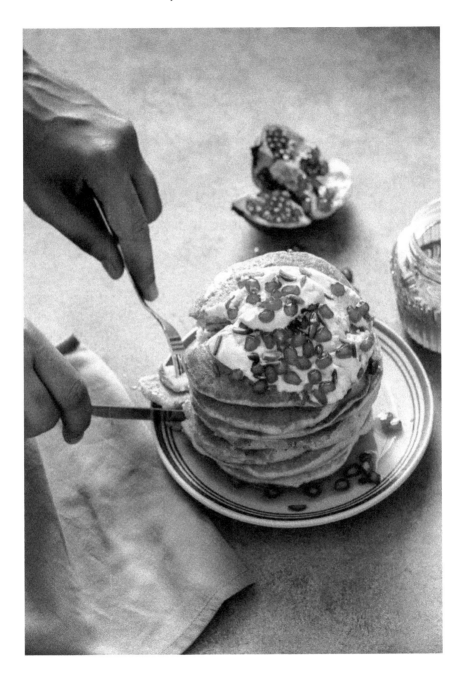

PLUMS PANCAKES

Serves: 4

Prep Time: 10   Minutes

Cook Time: 30   Minutes

Total Time: 40   Minutes

INGREDIENTS

-          1 cup whole wheat flour

-          ¼ tsp baking soda

-          ¼ tsp baking powder

-          1 cup plums

-          2 eggs

-          1 cup milk

DIRECTIONS

1. In a bowl combine all ingredients together and mix well

2. In a skillet heat olive oil

3. Pour ¼ of the batter and cook each pancake for 1-2 minutes per side

4. When ready remove from heat and serve

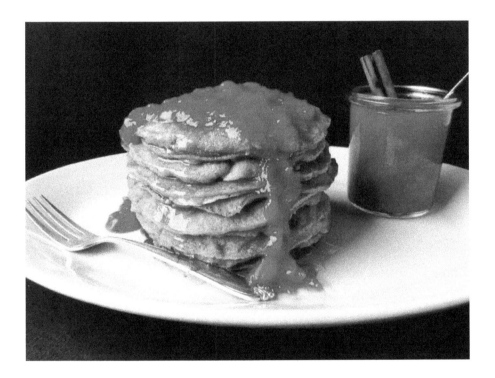

PLANTAIN MUFFINS

Serves: *8-12*

Prep Time: *10*   Minutes

Cook Time: *20*   Minutes

Total Time: *30*   Minutes

INGREDIENTS

- 2 eggs

- 1 tablespoon olive oil

- 1 cup milk

- 2 cups whole wheat flour

- 1 tsp baking soda

- ¼ tsp baking soda

- 1 tsp ginger

- 1 tsp cinnamon

- ¼ cup molasses

- 1 cup plantain

DIRECTIONS

1. In a bowl combine all wet ingredients

2. In another bowl combine all dry ingredients

3. Combine wet and dry ingredients together

4. Pour mixture into 8-12 prepared muffin cups, fill 2/3 of the cups

5. Bake for 18-20 minutes at 375 F

6. When ready remove from the oven and serve

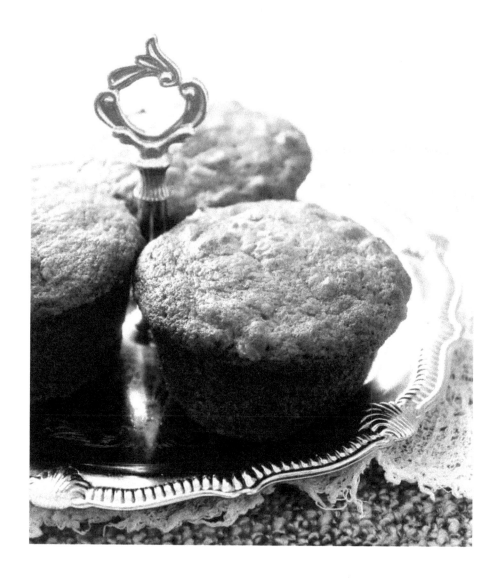

PEACHES MUFFINS

Serves: *8-12*

Prep Time: *10* Minutes

Cook Time: *20* Minutes

Total Time: *30* Minutes

INGREDIENTS

- 2 eggs

- 1 tablespoon olive oil

- 1 cup milk

- 2 cups whole wheat flour

- 1 tsp baking soda

- ¼ tsp baking soda

- 1 tsp cinnamon

- 1 cup peaches

DIRECTIONS

1. In a bowl combine all wet ingredients

2. In another bowl combine all dry ingredients

3. Combine wet and dry ingredients together

4. Pour mixture into 8-12 prepared muffin cups, fill 2/3 of the cups

5. Bake for 18-20 minutes at 375 F

6. When ready remove from the oven and serve

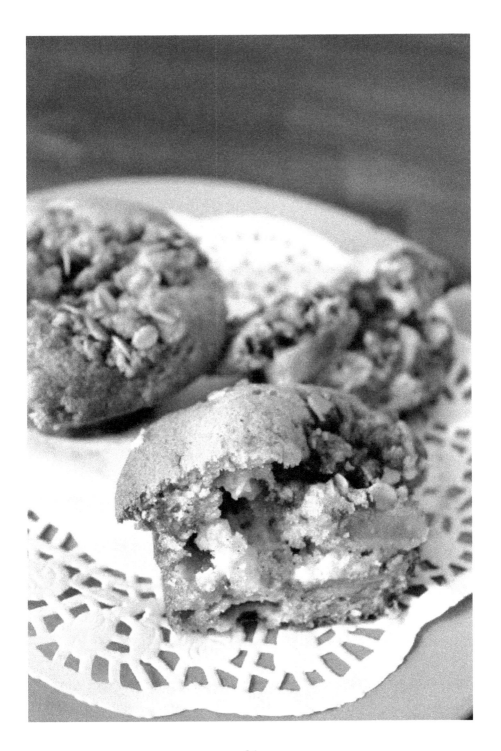

PEAR MUFFINS

Serves: *8-12*

Prep Time: *10*   Minutes

Cook Time: *20*   Minutes

Total Time: *30*   Minutes

INGREDIENTS

- 2 eggs

- 1 tablespoon olive oil

- 1 cup milk

- 2 cups whole wheat flour

- 1 tsp baking soda

- ¼ tsp baking soda

- 1 tsp cinnamon

- 1 cup pears

DIRECTIONS

1. In a bowl combine all wet ingredients

2. In another bowl combine all dry ingredients

3. Combine wet and dry ingredients together

4. Pour mixture into 8-12 prepared muffin cups, fill 2/3 of the cups

5. Bake for 18-20 minutes at 375 F

6. When ready remove from the oven and serve

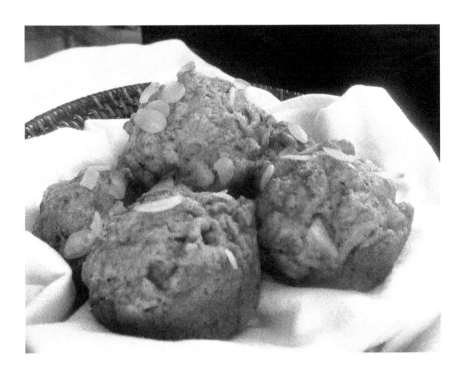

PAPAYA MUFFINS

Serves: *8-12*

Prep Time: *10* Minutes

Cook Time: *20* Minutes

Total Time: *30* Minutes

INGREDIENTS

- 2 eggs

- 1 tablespoon olive oil

- 1 cup milk

- 2 cups whole wheat flour

- 1 tsp baking soda

- ¼ tsp baking soda

- 1 tsp cinnamon

- 1 cup papaya

DIRECTIONS

1. In a bowl combine all wet ingredients

2. In another bowl combine all dry ingredients

3. Combine wet and dry ingredients together

4. Pour mixture into 8-12 prepared muffin cups, fill 2/3 of the cups

5. Bake for 18-20 minutes at 375 F

6. When ready remove from the oven and serv

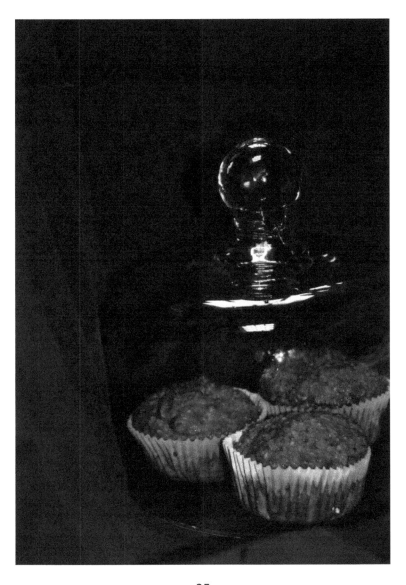

NECTARINE MUFFINS

Serves: 8-12

Prep Time: 10 Minutes

Cook Time: 20 Minutes

Total Time: 30 Minutes

INGREDIENTS

- 2 eggs

- 1 tablespoon olive oil

- 1 cup milk

- 2 cups whole wheat flour

- 1 tsp baking soda

- ¼ tsp baking soda

- 1 tsp cinnamon

- 1 cup nectarine

DIRECTIONS

1. In a bowl combine all wet ingredients

2. In another bowl combine all dry ingredients

3. Combine wet and dry ingredients together

4. Pour mixture into 8-12 prepared muffin cups, fill 2/3 of the cups

5. Bake for 18-20 minutes at 375 F

6. When ready remove from the oven and serve

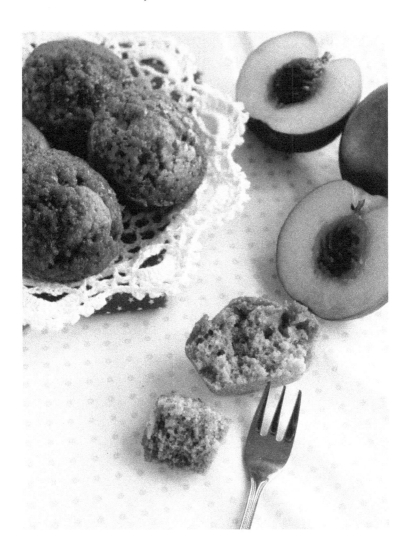

JUJUBE MUFFINS

Serves: *8-12*

Prep Time: *10* Minutes

Cook Time: *20* Minutes

Total Time: *30* Minutes

INGREDIENTS

- 2 eggs

- 1 tablespoon olive oil

- 1 cup milk

- 2 cups whole wheat flour

- 1 tsp baking soda

- ¼ tsp baking soda

- 1 tsp cinnamon

- 1 cup jujube

DIRECTIONS

1. In a bowl combine all wet ingredients

2. In another bowl combine all dry ingredients

3. Combine wet and dry ingredients together

4. Pour mixture into 8-12 prepared muffin cups, fill 2/3 of the cups

5. Bake for 18-20 minutes at 375 F

6. When ready remove from the oven and serve

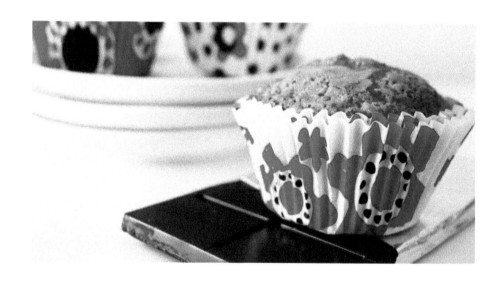

ARROWROOT OMELETTE

Serves: *1*

Prep Time: *5*   Minutes

Cook Time: *10*   Minutes

Total Time: *15*   Minutes

INGREDIENTS

- 2 eggs

- ¼ tsp salt

- ¼ tsp black pepper

- 1 tablespoon olive oil

- ¼ cup cheese

- ¼ tsp basil

- 1 cup arrowroot

DIRECTIONS

1. In a bowl combine all ingredients together and mix well

2. In a skillet heat olive oil and pour the egg mixture

3. Cook for 1-2 minutes per side

4. When ready remove omelette from the skillet and serve

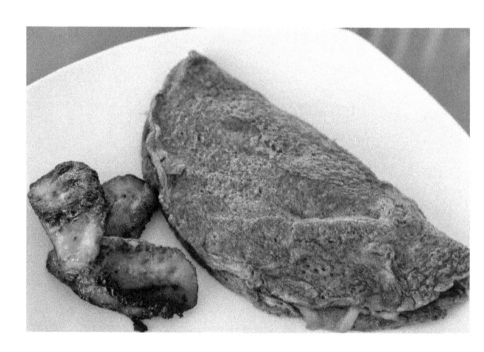

ARUGULA OMELETTE

Serves: *1*

Prep Time: *5*   Minutes

Cook Time: *10*   Minutes

Total Time: *15*   Minutes

INGREDIENTS

-        2 eggs

-        ¼ tsp salt

-        ¼ tsp black pepper

-        1 tablespoon olive oil

-        ¼ cup cheese

-        ¼ tsp basil

-        1 cup arugula

DIRECTIONS

1. In a bowl combine all ingredients together and mix well

2. In a skillet heat olive oil and pour the egg mixture

3. Cook for 1-2 minutes per side

4. When ready remove omelette from the skillet and serve

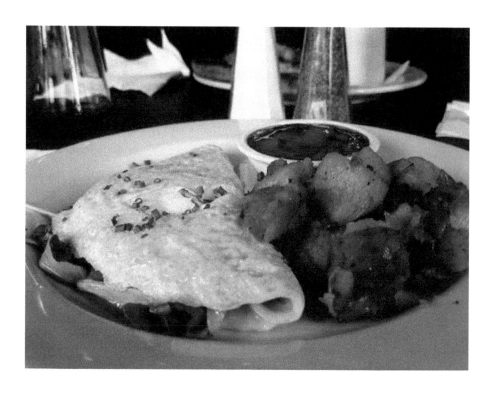

ARTICHOKE OMELETTE

Serves: *1*

Prep Time: *5* Minutes

Cook Time: *10* Minutes

Total Time: *15* Minutes

INGREDIENTS

- 2 eggs

- ¼ tsp salt

- ¼ tsp black pepper

- 1 tablespoon olive oil

- ¼ cup cheese

- ¼ tsp basil

- 1 cup artichoke

DIRECTIONS

1. In a bowl combine all ingredients together and mix well

2. In a skillet heat olive oil and pour the egg mixture

3. Cook for 1-2 minutes per side

4. When ready remove omelette from the skillet and serve

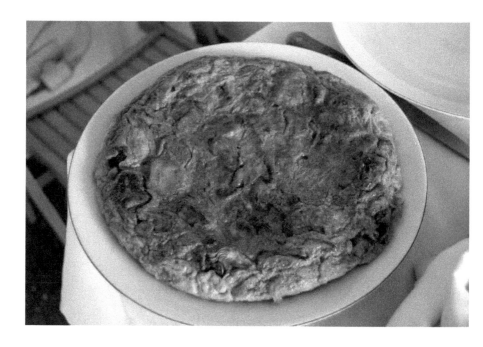

BEETS OMELETTE

Serves: *1*

Prep Time: *5* Minutes

Cook Time: *10* Minutes

Total Time: *15* Minutes

INGREDIENTS

- 2 eggs

- ¼ tsp salt

- ¼ tsp black pepper

- 1 tablespoon olive oil

- ¼ cup cheese

- ¼ tsp basil

- 1 cup beets

DIRECTIONS

1. In a bowl combine all ingredients together and mix well

2. In a skillet heat olive oil and pour the egg mixture

3. Cook for 1-2 minutes per side

4. When ready remove omelette from the skillet and serve

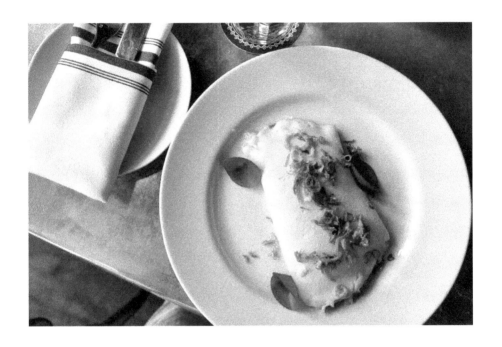

JICAMA OMELETTE

Serves: 1

Prep Time: 5   Minutes

Cook Time: 10   Minutes

Total Time: 15   Minutes

INGREDIENTS

-        2 eggs

-        ¼ tsp salt

-        ¼ tsp black pepper

-        1 tablespoon olive oil

-        ¼ cup cheese

-        ¼ tsp basil

-        1 cup jicama

DIRECTIONS

1. In a bowl combine all ingredients together and mix well

2. In a skillet heat olive oil and pour the egg mixture

3. Cook for 1-2 minutes per side

4. When ready remove omelette from the skillet and serve

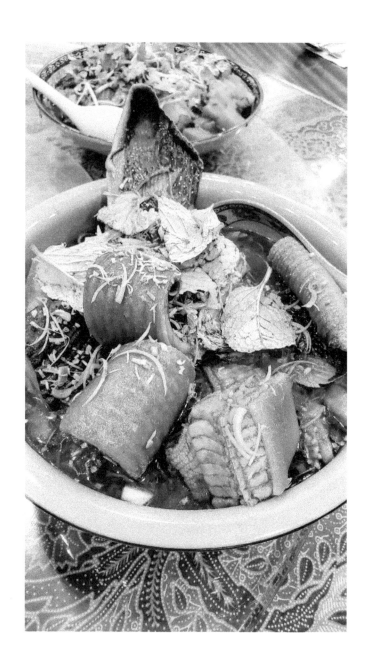

5 MINUTE BAKED EGGS

Serves: *2*

Prep Time: *5*   Minutes

Cook Time: *10*   Minutes

Total Time: *15*   Minutes

INGREDIENTS

- 1 tablespoon butter

- 1 tablespoon milk

- 2 eggs

- 1 tsp garlic powder

DIRECTIONS

1. Coat a baking dish with butter and milk

2. Crack the eggs in the baking dish, add garlic powder and broil for 6-7 minutes in the oven

3. When ready remove from the oven and serve

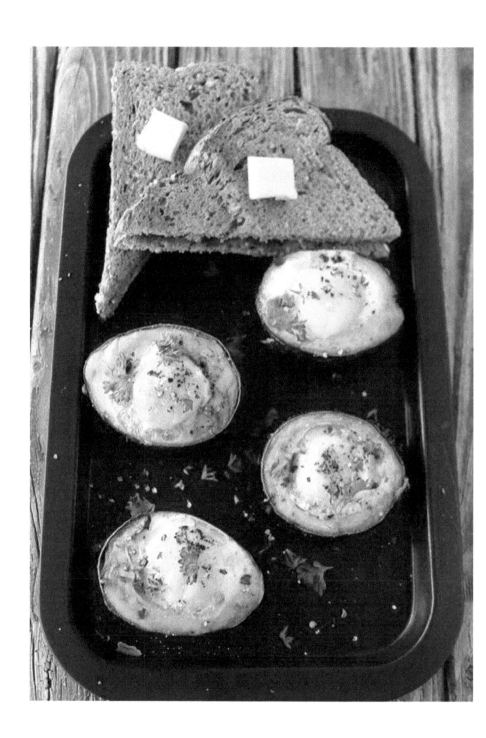

YOGURT PARFAIT

Serves: *1*

Prep Time: *5* Minutes

Cook Time: *5* Minutes

Total Time: *10* Minutes

INGREDIENTS

- ¼ cup yogurt

- ¼ cup pecans

- 1 tsp brewed coffee

DIRECTIONS

1. In a bowl combine coffee, pecans and yogurt

2. Add a pinch of cinnamon and serve

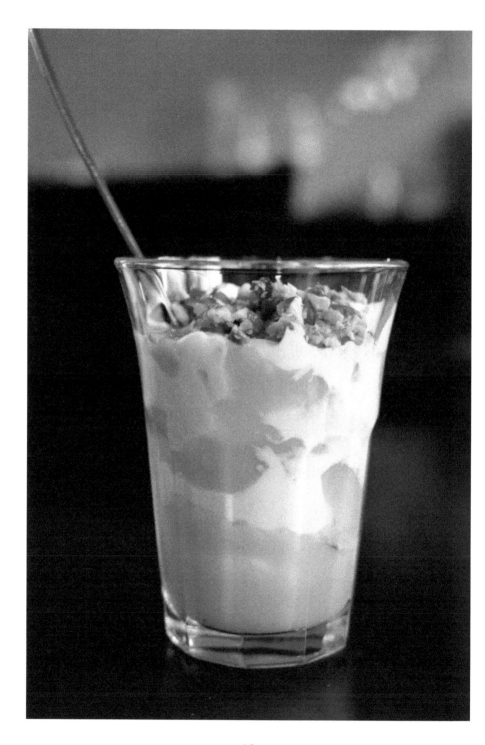

CINNAMON GRANOLA

Serves: *4-6*

Prep Time: *10*   Minutes

Cook Time: *20*   Minutes

Total Time: *30*   Minutes

INGREDIENTS

-        2 cups oats

-        ¼ cup coconut flakes

-        ¼ cup walnuts

-        1 tablespoon pumpkin seeds

-        ¼ tsp cinnamon

-        ¼ tsp nutmeg

-        ¼ cup honey

-        ¼ cup raisins

-        ¼ cup cranberries

DIRECTIONS

1. In a bowl combine pumpkin seeds, oats, walnuts, nutmeg, cinnamon and cranberries

2. Add honey, coconut flakes and mix well

3. Spread the mixture on a baking sheet

4. Bake at 325 F for 18-20 minutes

5. When ready remove from the oven and serve

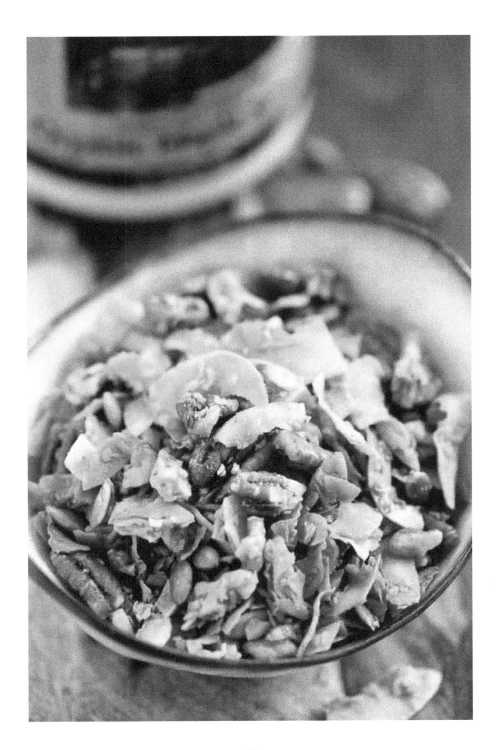

BANANA OVERNIGHT OATS

Serves: *1*

Prep Time: *5*   Minutes

Cook Time: *5*   Minutes

Total Time: *10*   Minutes

INGREDIENTS

-        1 cup oats

-        1 cup almond milk

-        1 banana

-        ½ Greek Yogurt

-        1 tablespoon coconut flakes

-        1 tablespoon honey

-        1 tablespoon chia seeds

-        1 tsp vanilla extract

DIRECTIONS

1. In a bowl combine all ingredients together and mix well

2. Divide mixture into 2-3-4 serving bowls and refrigerate

3. Serve in the morning

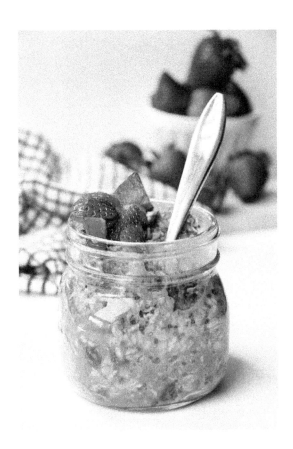

SIMPLE PIZZA RECIPE

Serves: *6-8*

Prep Time: *10*   Minutes

Cook Time: *15*   Minutes

Total Time: *25*   Minutes

INGREDIENTS

- 1 pizza crust

- ½ cup tomato sauce

- ¼ black pepper

- 1 cup pepperoni slices

- 1 cup mozzarella cheese

- 1 cup olives

DIRECTIONS

1. Spread tomato sauce on the pizza crust

2. Place all the toppings on the pizza crust

3. Bake the pizza at 425 F for 12-15 minutes

4. When ready remove pizza from the oven and serve

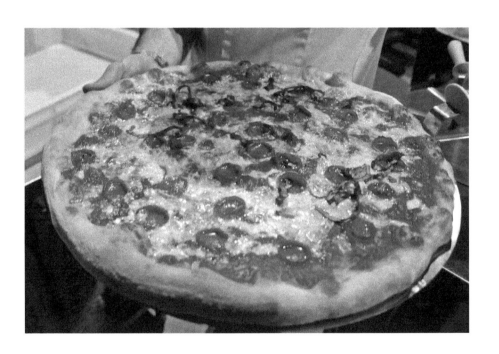

SUMMER EGGS

Serves: *2*

Prep Time: *10*   Minutes

Cook Time: *20*   Minutes

Total Time: *30*   Minutes

INGREDIENTS

-        2 tablespoons olive oil

-        1 lb. courgettes

-        ½ lb. cherry tomatoes

-        2 garlic cloves

-        3 eggs

DIRECTIONS

1. In a frying pan add courgettes and fry for 5-6 minutes

2. Add garlic, tomatoes and cook for another 2-3 minutes

3. Crack the eggs over and cover with a lid

4. Cook for another 6-7 minutes

5. When ready remove from heat and serve

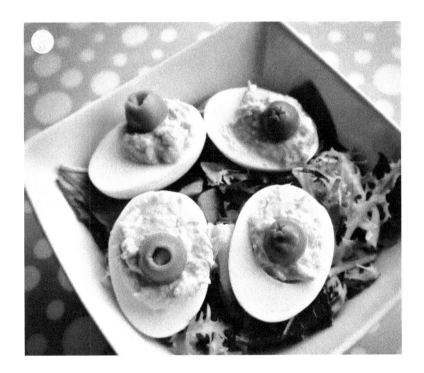

TACO SALAD

Serves: *2*

Prep Time: *5*   Minutes

Cook Time: *5*   Minutes

Total Time: *10*   Minutes

INGREDIENTS

- ½ cup olive oil

- 1 lb. cooked steak

- 1 tablespoon taco seasoning

- Juice of 1 lime

- 1 tsp cumin

- 1 head romaine lettuce

- 1 cup corn

- 1 cup beans

- 1 cup tomatoes

DIRECTIONS

1. In a bowl combine all ingredients together and mix well

2. Serve with dressing

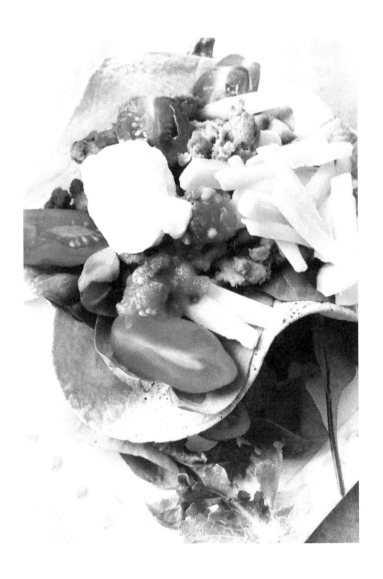

KALE SALAD

Serves: 2

Prep Time: 5 Minutes

Cook Time: 5 Minutes

Total Time: 10 Minutes

INGREDIENTS

- 2 cups kale

- 1 tablespoon hemp seeds

- 1 cucumber

- 1 tsp honey

- 1 tsp olive oil

- 1 handful parsley

DIRECTIONS

1. In a bowl combine all ingredients together and mix well

2. Serve with dressing

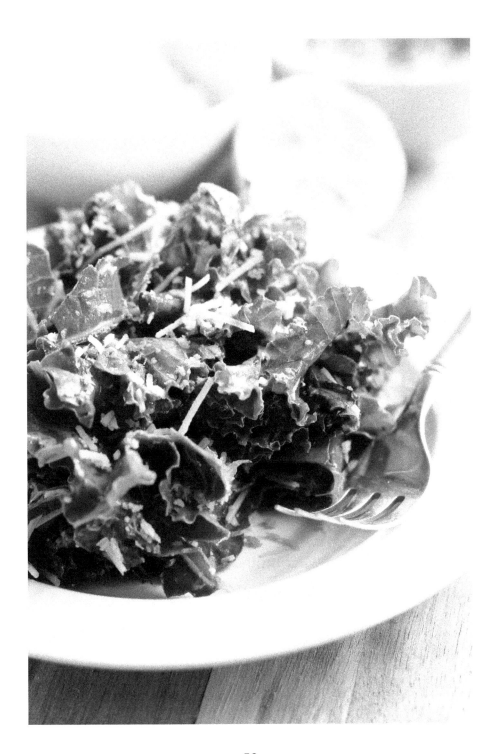

CHARRED SALAD

Serves: 2

Prep Time: 5 Minutes

Cook Time: 5 Minutes

Total Time: 10 Minutes

INGREDIENTS

- 2 tablespoons olive oil

- 1 shallot

- 2 cups cooked corn

- 1 red Chile

- 4 tablespoons lemon juice

- ¼ cup parmesan cheese

DIRECTIONS

1. In a bowl combine all ingredients together and mix well

2. Serve with dressing

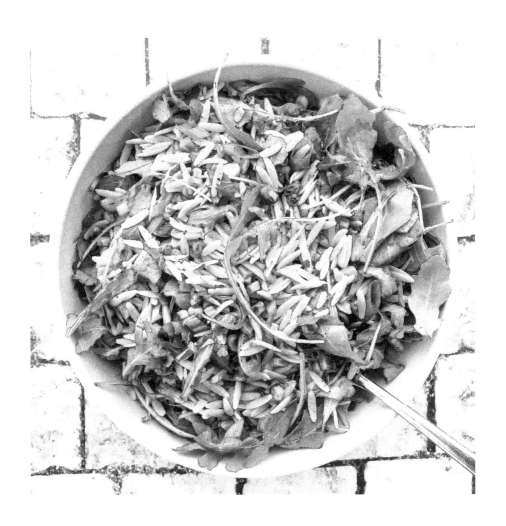

CUCUMBER SALAD

Serves: *2*

Prep Time: *5*   Minutes

Cook Time: *5*   Minutes

Total Time: *10*   Minutes

INGREDIENTS

- 4-5 cucumbers

- ¼ red onion

- 1 tsp salt

- 1 tsp sugar

- 1 tsp vinegar

- 1 cup veggies

- 3-4 mint leaves

DIRECTIONS

1. In a bowl combine all ingredients together and mix well

2. Serve with dressing

FIG CAPRESE SALAD

Serves: 2

Prep Time: 5   Minutes

Cook Time: 5   Minutes

Total Time: 10   Minutes

INGREDIENTS

-        1 cup mozzarella

-        1 cup figs

-        3-4 basil leaves

-        2 tablespoons olive oil

DIRECTIONS

1. In a bowl combine all ingredients together and mix well

2. Serve with dressing

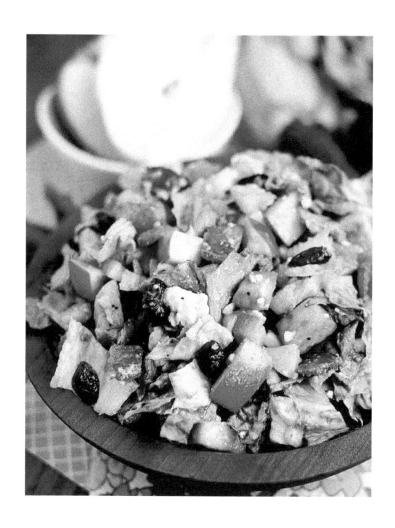

STEAK SALAD

Serves: *2*

Prep Time: *5* Minutes

Cook Time: *5* Minutes

Total Time: *10* Minutes

INGREDIENTS

- 1 lb. steak

- 1 shallot

- 1 tablespoon wine vinegar

- 4 tablespoons olive oil

- 1 cup cherry tomatoes

- 1 cucumber

- 1 head lettuce

- ½ avocado

DIRECTIONS

1. In a bowl combine all ingredients together and mix well

2. Serve with dressing

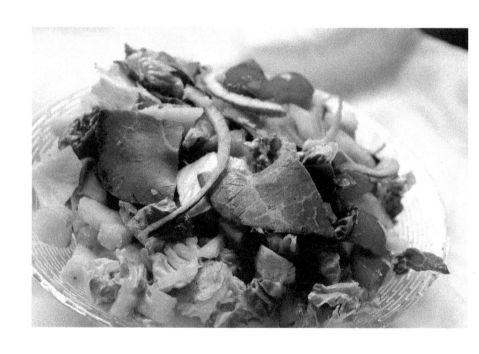

QUESO FRESCO SALAD

Serves: *2*

Prep Time: *5*   Minutes

Cook Time: *5*   Minutes

Total Time: *10*   Minutes

INGREDIENTS

- ¼ cup olive oil

- 2 sliced pitas

- 2 tablespoons lemon juice

- 1 romaine heart

- 1 onion

- 1 cucumber

- 1 cup cherry tomatoes

- 1 cup cilantro

- ¼ cup parsley

- 4-5 oz. queso fresco

DIRECTIONS

1. In a bowl combine all ingredients together and mix well

2. Serve with dressing

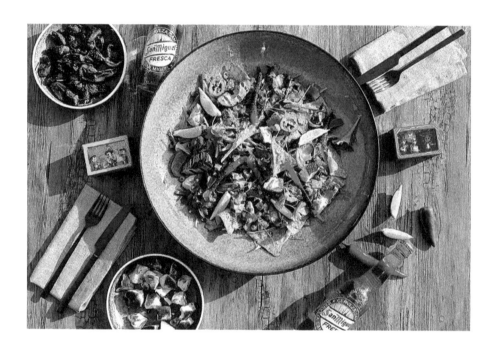

PEPPER PASTA SALAD

Serves: 2

Prep Time: 5   Minutes

Cook Time: 5   Minutes

Total Time: 10   Minutes

INGREDIENTS

-         ¼ cup hazelnuts

-         ½ cup pistachios

-         ¼ cup almonds

-         2 lb. bell peppers

-         ¼ cup olive oil

-         1 head garlic

-         2 sprigs thyme

-         1 lb. rigatoni

-         4 oz. ricotta

-         1 cup basil leaves

DIRECTIONS

1. In a bowl combine all ingredients together and mix well

2. Serve with dressing

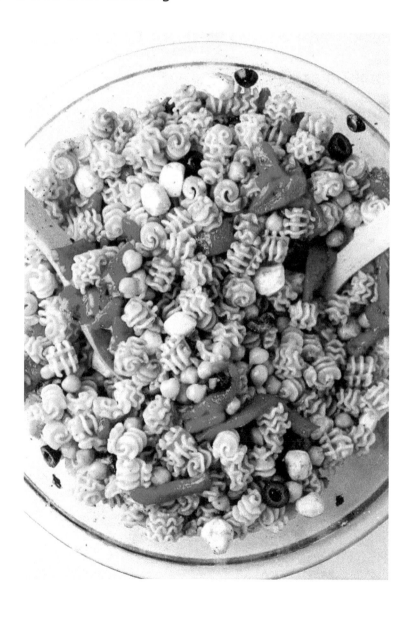

COBB SALAD

Serves: 2

Prep Time: 5   Minutes

Cook Time: 5   Minutes

Total Time: 10   Minutes

INGREDIENTS

-        6 tablespoons olive oil

-        3 garlic cloves

-        2 cooked chicken things

-        1 tsp curry powder

-        1 tsp lemon juice

-        1 avocado

-        1 mango

-        1 cup tomatoes

DIRECTIONS

1. In a bowl combine all ingredients together and mix well

2. Serve with dressing

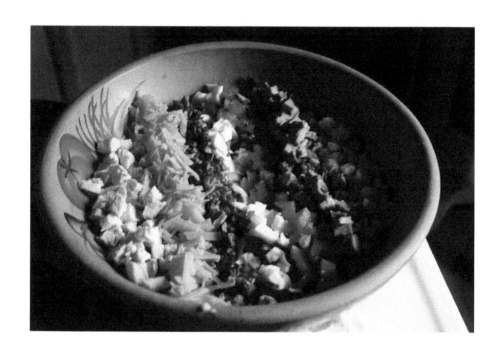

RADICCHIO SALAD

Serves: *2*

Prep Time: *5*   Minutes

Cook Time: *5*   Minutes

Total Time: *10* Minutes

INGREDIENTS

- ¼ cup hazelnuts

- ¼ cup walnuts

- 2 nectarines

- 2 radicchios

- 2 scallions

- ¼ cup parsley

- ¼ cup olive oil

- ¼ cup cheese

DIRECTIONS

1. In a bowl combine all ingredients together and mix well

2. Serve with dressing

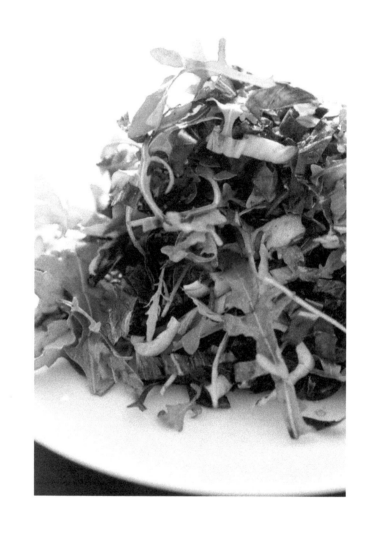

ZUCCHINI PIZZA

Serves: *6-8*

Prep Time: *10* Minutes

Cook Time: *15* Minutes

Total Time: *25* Minutes

INGREDIENTS

- 1 pizza crust

- ½ cup tomato sauce

- ¼ black pepper

- 1 cup zucchini slices

- 1 cup mozzarella cheese

- 1 cup olives

DIRECTIONS

1. Spread tomato sauce on the pizza crust

2. Place all the toppings on the pizza crust

3. Bake the pizza at 425 F for 12-15 minutes

4. When ready remove pizza from the oven and serve

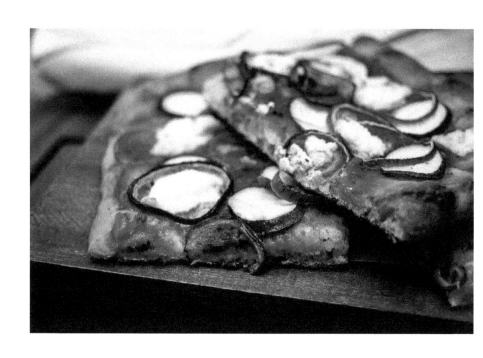

LENTIL FRITATTA

Serves: *2*

Prep Time: *10* Minutes

Cook Time: *20* Minutes

Total Time: *30* Minutes

INGREDIENTS

- ½ lb. lentil

- 1 tablespoon olive oil

- ½ red onion

- ¼ tsp salt

- 2 eggs

- 2 oz. cheddar cheese

- 1 garlic clove

- ¼ tsp dill

DIRECTIONS

1. In a bowl whisk eggs with salt and cheese

2. In a frying pan heat olive oil and pour egg mixture

3. Add remaining ingredients and mix well

4. Serve when ready

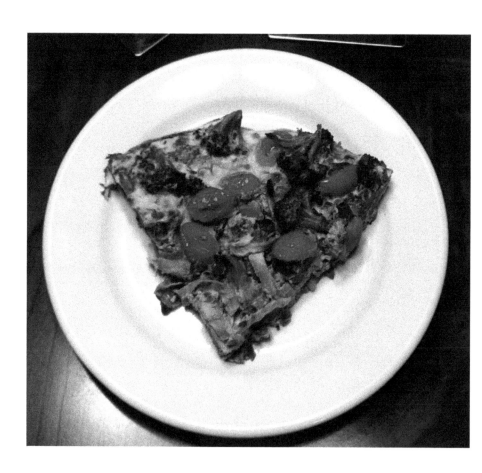

SPINACH FRITATTA

Serves: *2*

Prep Time: *10*   Minutes

Cook Time: *20*   Minutes

Total Time: *30*   Minutes

INGREDIENTS

-         ½ lb. spinach

-         1 tablespoon olive oil

-         ½ red onion

-         2 eggs

-         ¼ tsp salt

-         2 oz. cheddar cheese

-         1 garlic clove

-         ¼ tsp dill

DIRECTIONS

1. In a skillet sauté spinach until tender

2. In a bowl whisk eggs with salt and cheese

3. In a frying pan heat olive oil and pour egg mixture

4. Add remaining ingredients and mix well

5. When ready serve with sautéed spinach

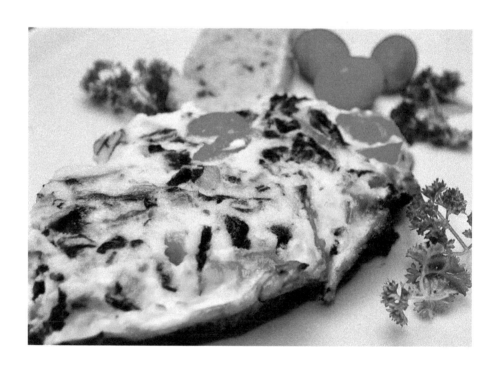

BLACK BEAN FRITATTA

Serves: *2*

Prep Time: *10* Minutes

Cook Time: *20* Minutes

Total Time: *30* Minutes

INGREDIENTS

-        1 cup cooked black beans

-        1 tablespoon olive oil

-        ½ red onion

-        ¼ tsp salt

-        2 oz. cheddar cheese

-        1 garlic clove

-        ¼ tsp dill

-        2 eggs

DIRECTIONS

1. In a bowl whisk eggs with salt and cheese

2. In a frying pan heat olive oil and pour egg mixture

3. Add remaining ingredients and mix well

4. Serve when ready

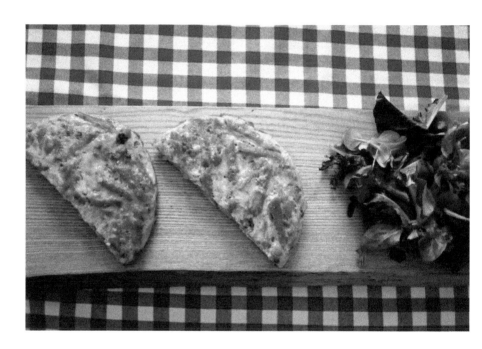

CHEESE FRITATTA

Serves: 2

Prep Time: 10 Minutes

Cook Time: 20 Minutes

Total Time: 30 Minutes

INGREDIENTS

- 1 tablespoon olive oil

- ½ red onion

- ¼ tsp salt

- 2 oz. cheddar cheese

- 1 garlic clove

- ¼ tsp dill

- 2 eggs

DIRECTIONS

1. In a bowl combine cheddar cheese and onion

2. In a frying pan heat olive oil and pour egg mixture

3. Add remaining ingredients and mix well

4. Serve when ready

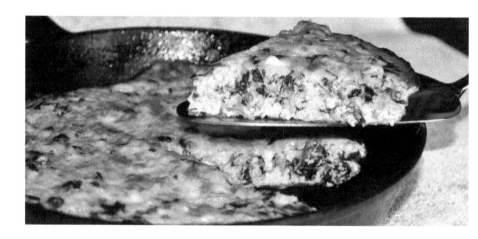

BROCCOLI FRITATTA

Serves: *2*

Prep Time: *10*   Minutes

Cook Time: *20*   Minutes

Total Time: *30*   Minutes

INGREDIENTS

- 1 cup broccoli

- 1 tablespoon olive oil

- ½ red onion

- ¼ tsp salt

- 2 oz. cheddar cheese

- 1 garlic clove

- 2 eggs

- ¼ tsp dill

DIRECTIONS

1. In a skillet sauté broccoli until tender

2. In a bowl whisk eggs with salt and cheese

3. In a frying pan heat olive oil and pour egg mixture

4. Add remaining ingredients and mix well

5. When ready serve with sautéed broccoli

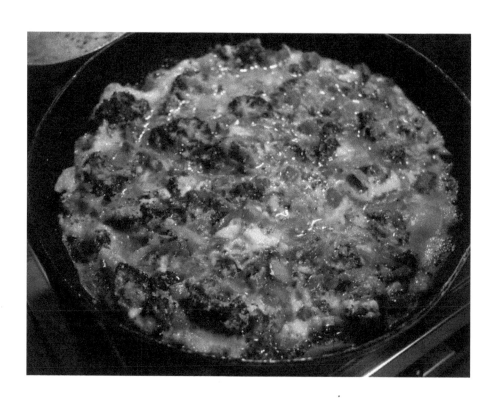

SHAKSHUKA

Serves: *2*

Prep Time: *10*   Minutes

Cook Time: *20*   Minutes

Total Time: *30*   Minutes

INGREDIENTS

-      1 tablespoon olive oil

-      1 red onion

-      1 red chili

-      1 garlic clove

-      2 cans cherry tomatoes

-      2 eggs

DIRECTIONS

1. In a frying pan cook garlic, chili, onions until soft

2. Stir in tomatoes and cook until mixture thickens

3. Crack the eggs over the sauce

4. Cover with a lid and cook for another 7-8 minutes

5. When ready remove from heat and serve

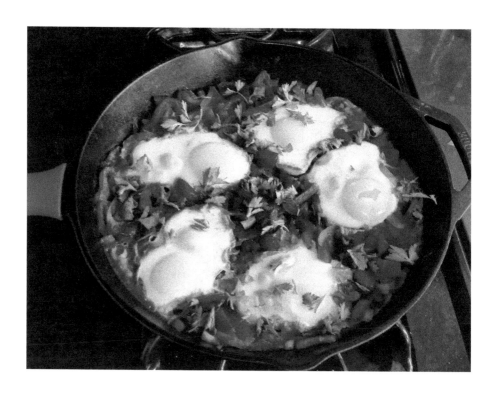

BACON-SALMON

Serves: 2

Prep Time: 10 Minutes

Cook Time: 20 Minutes

Total Time: 30 Minutes

INGREDIENTS

- 2 filets salmon

- 2 slices bacon

- 1 tablespoon olive oil

- Lemon wedges

DIRECTIONS

1. Wrap the bacon around the salmon fillets

2. Place the fillets in a baking dish

3. Drizzle olive oil and add lemon wedges

4. Bake at 350 F for 18-20 minutes

5. When ready remove from the oven and serve

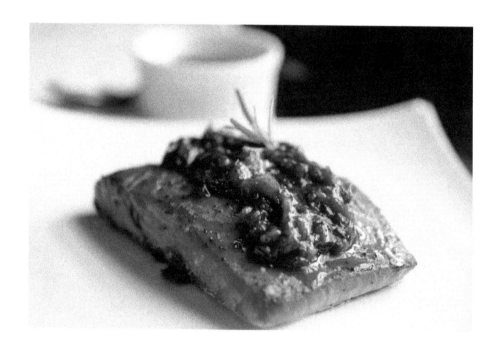

SLOW COOKER CHICKEN

Serves: *2*

Prep Time: *10*   Minutes

Cook Time: *8*   Hours

Total Time: *8*   Hours 10 Minutes

INGREDIENTS

- 4 chicken breasts

- 8 slices bacon

- 1 tablespoon oregano

- 1 tablespoon rosemary

- 4 tablespoons olive oil

DIRECTIONS

1. Place all the ingredients in a slow cooker

2. Cook on low heat for 7-8 hours

3. When ready remove from the slow cooker and serve

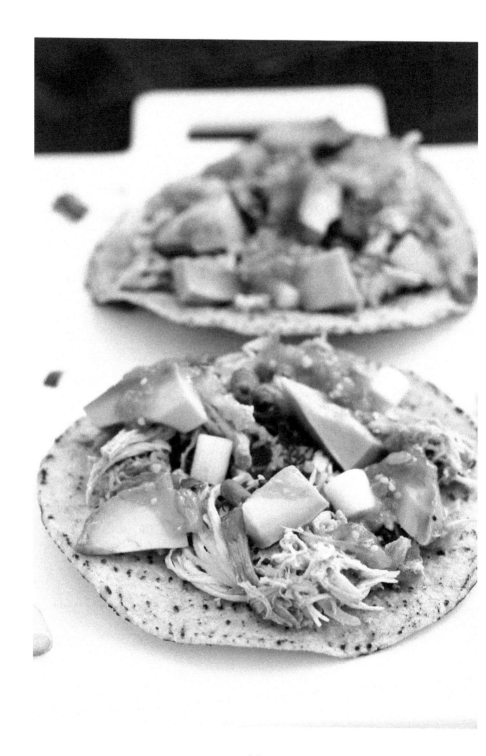

GRILLED FLANK STEAK

Serves: 4-6

Prep Time: 10   Minutes

Cook Time: 30   Minutes

Total Time: 40   Minutes

INGREDIENTS

-         2 lbs. flank steak

-         1 cup olive oil

-         1 cup apple cider vinegar

-         Juice from 1 lemon

-         4 garlic cloves

-         1 tsp smoked paprika

-         1 tablespoon onion powder

-         1 tsp dried thyme

DIRECTIONS

1. In a bowl combine all ingredients together for the marinade

2. Cut steak into pieces and place in the marinade

3. Let the steak marinade overnight

4. Place the steak on the grill and cook for 3-4 minutes per side

5. When ready remove from the grill and serve

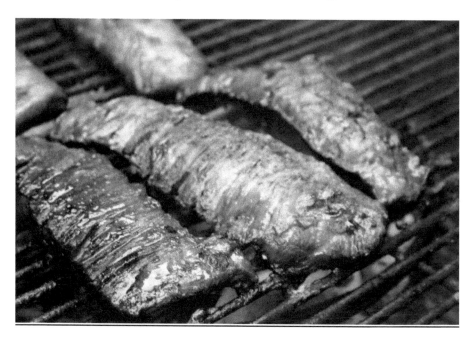

CHEESE MACARONI

Serves: *1*

Prep Time: *10* Minutes

Cook Time: *20* Minutes

Total Time: *30* Minutes

INGREDIENTS

- 1 lb. macaroni

- 1 cup cheddar cheese

- 1 cup Monterey Jack cheese

- 1 cup mozzarella cheese

- ¼ tsp salt

- ¼ tsp pepper

DIRECTIONS

1. In a pot bring water to a boil

2. Add pasta and cook until al dente

3. In a bowl combine all cheese together and add it to the pasta

4. When ready transfer to a bowl, add salt, pepper and serve

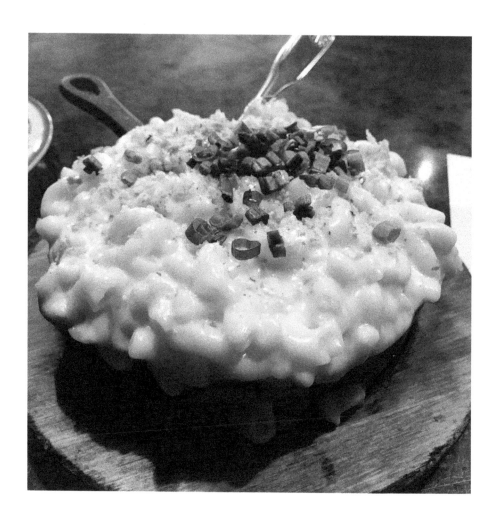

POTATO CASSEROLE

Serves: *2*

Prep Time: *10* Minutes

Cook Time: *20* Minutes

Total Time: *30* Minutes

INGREDIENTS

- 5-6 large potatoes

- ¼ cup sour cream

- ½ cup butter

- 5-6 bacon strips

- 1-2 cups mozzarella cheese

- ¼ cup heavy cream

DIRECTIONS

1. Place the potatoes in a pot with boiling water, cook until tender

2. Place the potatoes in a bowl, add sour cream, butter, cheese and mix well

3. In a baking dish place the bacon strips and cover with potato mixture

4. Add remaining mozzarella cheese on top

5. Bake at 325 F for 15-18 minutes or until the mozzarella is fully melted

6. When ready remove from the oven and serve

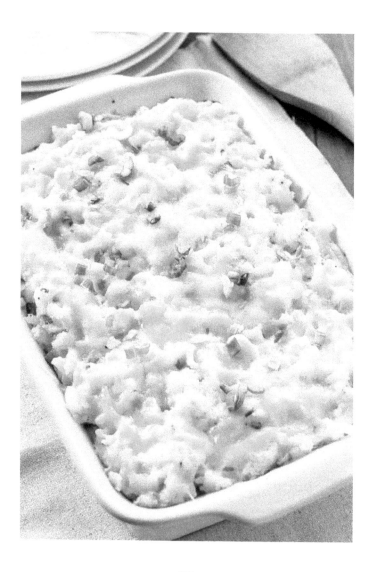

CHEESE STUFFED SHELLS

Serves: *2*

Prep Time: *10* Minutes

Cook Time: *30* Minutes

Total Time: *40* Minutes

INGREDIENTS

- 2-3 cups macaroni

- 2 cups cream cheese

- 1 cup spaghetti sauce

- 1 cup onions

- 1 cup mozzarella cheese

DIRECTIONS

1. In a pot boil water and add shells

2. Cook for 12-15 minutes

3. In a baking dish add spaghetti sauce

4. In a bowl combine cream cheese, onion and set aside

5. Add cream cheese to the shells and place them into the baking dish

6. Bake at 325 F for 30 minutes or until golden brown

7. When ready remove from the oven and serve

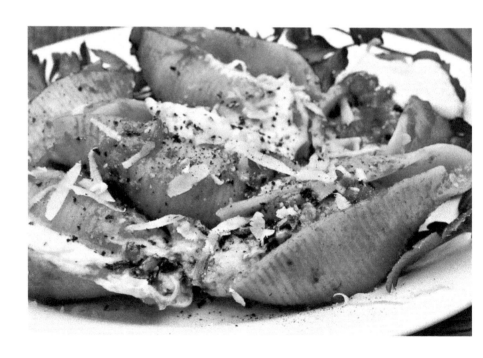

POTATO SOUP

Serves: *4-6*

Prep Time: *10* Minutes

Cook Time: *50* Minutes

Total Time: *60* Minutes

INGREDIENTS

- 1 onion

- 2-3 carrots

- 2 tablespoons flour

- 5-6 large potatoes

- 2 cups milk

- 2 cups bouillon

- 1 cup water

- 2 cups milk

- 1 tsp salt

- 1 tsp pepper

DIRECTIONS

1. In a saucepan melt butter and sauce carrots, garlic and onion for 4-5 minutes

2. Add flour, milk, potatoes, bouillon and cook for another 15-20 minutes

3. Add pepper and remaining ingredients and cook on low heat for 20-30 minutes

4. When ready remove from heat and serve

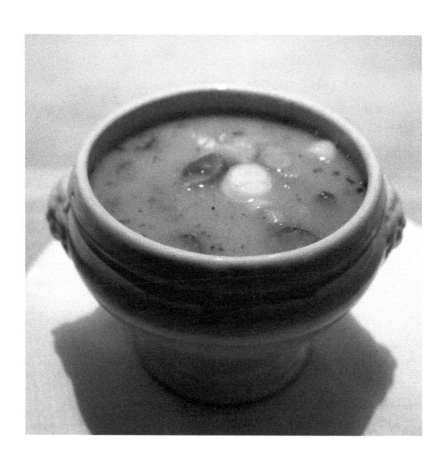

CHICKEN ALFREDO

Serves: *2*

Prep Time: *10*   Minutes

Cook Time: *20*   Minutes

Total Time: *30*   Minutes

INGREDIENTS

- 2-3 chicken breasts

- 1 lb. rotini

- 1 cup parmesan cheese

- 1 cup olive oil

- 1 tsp salt

- 1 tsp black pepper

- 1 tsp parsley

DIRECTIONS

1. In a pot add the rotini and cook on low heat for 12-15 minutes

2. In a frying pan heat olive oil, add chicken, salt, parsley, and cook until the chicken is brown

3. Drain the rotini and place the rotini in pan with chicken

4. Cook for 2-3 minutes

5. When ready remove from heat and serve with parmesan cheese on top

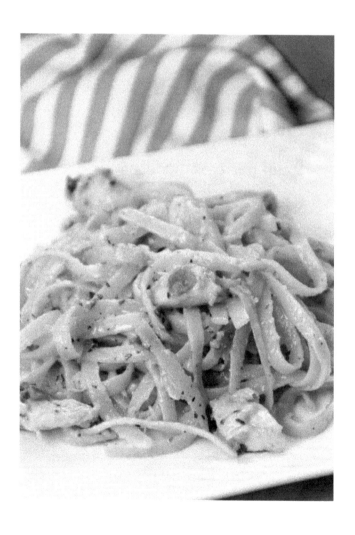

BUTTERNUT SQUASH PIZZA

Serves: *4-6*

Prep Time: *10*   Minutes

Cook Time: *15*   Minutes

Total Time: *25*   Minutes

INGREDIENTS

- 2 cups butternut squash

- ¼ tsp salt

- 1 pizza crust

- 5-6 tablespoons alfredo sauce

- 1 tsp olive oil

- 4-5 cups baby spinach

- 2-3 oz. goat cheese

DIRECTIONS

1. Place the pizza crust on a baking dish and spread the alfredo sauce

2. In a skillet sauté spinach and place it over the pizza crust

3. Add goat cheese, butternut squash, olive oil and salt

4. Bake pizza at 425 F for 8-10 minutes

5. When ready remove from the oven and serve

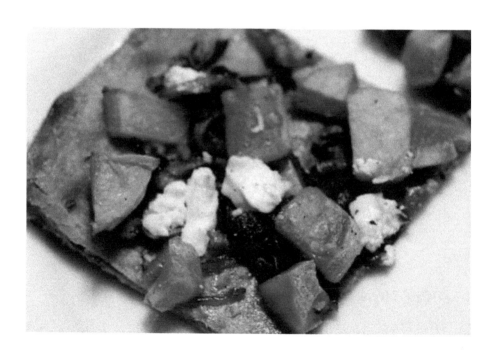

PENNE WITH ASPARAGUS

Serves: *2*

Prep Time: *10* Minutes

Cook Time: *20* Minutes

Total Time: *30* Minutes

INGREDIENTS

- 6-7 oz. penne pasta

- 2-3 bacon slices

- ¼ cup red onion

- 2 cups asparagus

- 1 cup chicken broth

- 2-3 cups spinach leaves

- ¼ cup parmesan cheese

DIRECTIONS

1. Cook pasta until al dente

2. In a skillet cook bacon until crispy and set aside

3. In a pan add onion, asparagus, broth and cook on low heat for 5-10 minutes

4. Add spinach, cheese, pepper, pasta and cook for another 5-6 minutes

5. When ready sprinkle bacon and serve

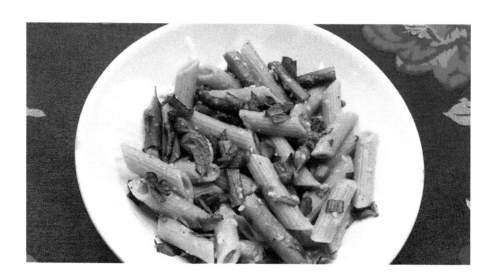

NOODLE SOUP

Serves: *4*

Prep Time: *10* Minutes

Cook Time: *20* Minutes

Total Time: *30* Minutes

INGREDIENTS

-       2-3 cups water

-       1 can chicken broth

-       1 tablespoon olive oil

-       ¼ red onion

-       ¼ cup celery

-       ¼ tsp salt

-       ¼ tsp black pepper

-       5-6 oz. fusilli pasta

-        2 cups chicken breast

-       2 tablespoons parsley

DIRECTIONS

1. In a pot boil water with broth

2. In a saucepan heat oil, add carrot, pepper, celery, onion, salt and sauté until tender

3. Add broth mixture to the mixture and pasta

4. Cook until al dente and stir in chicken breast, cook until chicken breast is tender

5. When ready remove from heat, stir in parsley and serve

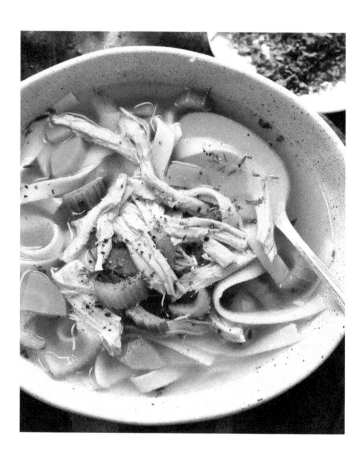

Lightning Source UK Ltd.
Milton Keynes UK
UKHW020746250621
386136UK00005B/57